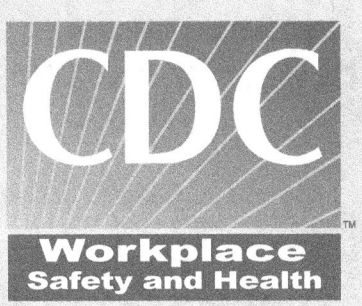

Evaluation of Isocyanate Exposure during Polyurethane Foam Application and Silica Exposure during Rock Dusting at an Underground Coal Mine

Kenneth W. Fent, PhD

Chad H. Dowell, MS, CIH

Health Hazard Evaluation Report
HETA 2009-0085-3107
Consolidation Coal Company
Blacksville, West Virginia
April 2010

Department of Health and Human Services
Centers for Disease Control and Prevention

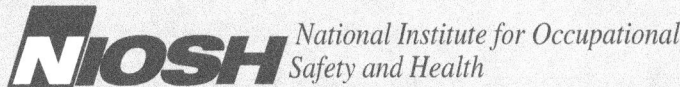

National Institute for Occupational
Safety and Health

The employer shall post a copy of this report for a period of 30 calendar days at or near the workplace(s) of affected employees. The employer shall take steps to insure that the posted determinations are not altered, defaced, or covered by other material during such period. [37 FR 23640, November 7, 1972, as amended at 45 FR 2653, January 14, 1980].

CONTENTS

REPORT

Abbreviations ii

Highlights of the NIOSH Health Hazard Evaluation............ iii

Summary v

Introduction.. 1

Assessment 3

Results & Dicussion.. 4

Conclusions 8

Recommendations... 9

References 12

APPENDIX A

Occupational Exposure Limits and Health Effects............. 14

ACKNOWLEDGMENTS

Acknowledgments and Availability of Report................... 19

ABBREVIATIONS

µg/m3	Micrograms per cubic meter
ACGIH®	American Conference of Governmental Industrial Hygienists
APF	Assigned protection factor
CFR	Code of Federal Regulations
HHE	Health hazard evaluation
IARC	International Agency for Research on Cancer
MDC	Minimum detectable concentration
MDI	Methylene diphenyl isocyanate
mmHg	Millimeters of mercury
MQC	Minimum quantifiable concentration
MSHA	Mine Safety and Health Administration
NAICS	North American Industry Classification System
ND	Nondetectable
NIOSH	National Institute for Occupational Safety and Health
OEL	Occupational exposure limit
OSHA	Occupational Safety and Health Administration
PAPR	Powered air purifying respirator
PBZ	Personal breathing zone
PEL	Permissible exposure limit
PPE	Personal protective equipment
PVC	Polyvinyl chloride
REL	Recommended exposure limit
STEL	Short-term exposure limit
TLV®	Threshold limit value
TWA	Time-weighted average
WEEL	Workplace environmental exposure level

HIGHLIGHTS OF THE NIOSH HEALTH HAZARD EVALUATION

The National Institute for Occupational Safety and Health (NIOSH) received a request for a health hazard evaluation (HHE) from the United Mine Workers of America, Local 1702. The request concerned potential methylene diphenyl isocyanate (MDI) exposure during the application of polyurethane foam and silica and asbestos exposures during rock dusting at the Consolidation Coal Company Blacksville #2 Mine in Blacksville, West Virginia.

What NIOSH Did

- We evaluated the mine on March 31, 2009, and September 14–17, 2009.
- We watched employees apply polyurethane foam and spray rock dust.
- We tested the surface of the foam applicator gun to see if it was contaminated with MDI.
- We took samples of the rock dust and analyzed them for silica and asbestos.
- We monitored the rock duster's breathing zone air for respirable silica and dust.

What NIOSH Found

- The foam applicator gun was not contaminated with MDI after spraying.
- The nitrile gloves the bratticeman wore while applying the foam protected his skin from MDI. Employees are unlikely to be exposed to MDI in the air. It does not readily evaporate at room temperature, and the foam was not aerosolized during application.
- We did not find asbestos in the rock dust, but we did find silica. The rock dusters' exposures to silica were below applicable exposure limits. However, statistical analysis showed that rock dusters are likely overexposed to silica some of the time.
- The bratticeman wore an appropriate respirator during foam application. The rock dusters wore appropriate respirators during most rock dusting activities. However, the mine did not have a written respiratory protection plan.

What Managers Can Do

- Continue to require bratticemen to wear nitrile gloves while applying polyurethane foam. Ensure that airflow in the mine carries rock dust away from the rock dusters.
- Require the use of respirators during rock dusting that are at least as protective as half-mask N95 filtering facepiece respirators.
- Implement a written respiratory protection program. The program should include medical evaluations, respirator fit testing, and periodic air monitoring.

What Employees Can Do

- Follow the Blacksville #2 Mine "Safe Work Instructions."

- Wear nitrile gloves while applying polyurethane foam, and discard these gloves after each use. Once leather gloves are used for foam application, they should not be used for other processes or worn over bare skin.

- Tell management about any health and safety concerns you may have.

- Take part in the labor-management health and safety committee.

SUMMARY

We found no evidence that the skin of the bratticemen was exposed to MDI during polyurethane foam application. The rock dusters' silica exposures we measured in air were below OELs. However, statistical analysis showed they are likely overexposed to silica some of the time. We recommended that bratticemen wear nitrile gloves, that rock dusters wear respirators at least as protective as half-mask N95 filtering facepiece respirators, and that rock dust be applied in well-ventilated areas. The mine should also implement a written respiratory protection program that incorporates medical evaluations and respirator fit testing.

NIOSH received a request for an HHE from the United Mine Workers of America, Local 1702 representing employees at the Consolidation Coal Company Blacksville #2 Mine in Blacksville, West Virginia. The HHE request concerned potential exposure to MDI during the application of polyurethane foam and exposure to silica and asbestos during rock dusting.

In an initial evaluation on March 31, 2009, we sampled the surface of the foam applicator gun for MDI contamination and collected bulk samples of the rock dust for silica and asbestos analysis. During a second evaluation on September 14–17, 2009, we collected PBZ air samples on day-shift rock dusters for respirable silica and dust.

We did not detect MDI on the surface of the foam applicator gun. The bratticeman who applied the foam wore nitrile gloves that protected his skin from MDI. Inhalation exposure to MDI is unlikely because the foam was not aerosolized during application and does not readily evaporate due to its low vapor pressure.

Low levels of silica were found in bulk samples of rock dust. Asbestos was not present in the rock dust. The PBZ air concentrations of respirable silica were below applicable OELs. However, according to a statistical analysis, there is a 73% probability that the rock dusters' PBZ concentrations may exceed the ACGIH TLV 5% of the time.

Because of the potential for overexposure to respirable silica, we recommend continued use of N95 filtering facepiece respirators. Additionally, the company should implement a written respiratory protection program that incorporates medical evaluations and respirator fit testing.

Keywords: NAICS 212112 (Bituminous Coal Underground Mining), silica, asbestos, calcium carbonate, isocyanates, MDI, rock dust, polyurethane foam, respirable dust

This page intentionally left blank.

On February 6, 2009, NIOSH received a request for an HHE from the United Mine Workers of America, Local 1702. The request concerned potential isocyanate exposures during polyurethane foam application and potential silica and asbestos exposures during rock dusting at the Consolidation Coal Company, Blacksville #2 Mine. On March 31, 2009, and September 14–17, 2009, we evaluated employee exposures to isocyanates, silica, dust, and asbestos.

Process Description

The Blacksville #2 Mine is a longwall bituminous coal mine between 500 and 900 feet underground. The mine opened in 1969, and approximately 10 square miles have been mined. Outdoor air is drawn into the mine using nine exhaust fans situated at various locations throughout the mine. At the time of the evaluation, 560 employees worked at the mine over three shifts. We evaluated two processes in the Blacksville #2 Mine, the application of polyurethane foam and rock dusting.

Bratticemen apply polyurethane foam to steel ventilation stoppings that block and direct airflow throughout the mine (Figure 1). The foam consists of Component A, containing monomeric and polymeric MDI, and Component B, containing a mixture of polyols. When Components A and B mix in the nozzle of the foam applicator gun, the MDI and polyols react rapidly to form polyurethane foam. The foam dries to touch in less than a minute and provides an impervious air seal. After application, the disposable nozzle is discarded, and petroleum jelly is applied to the gun face and valve stems before the applicator gun is stored.

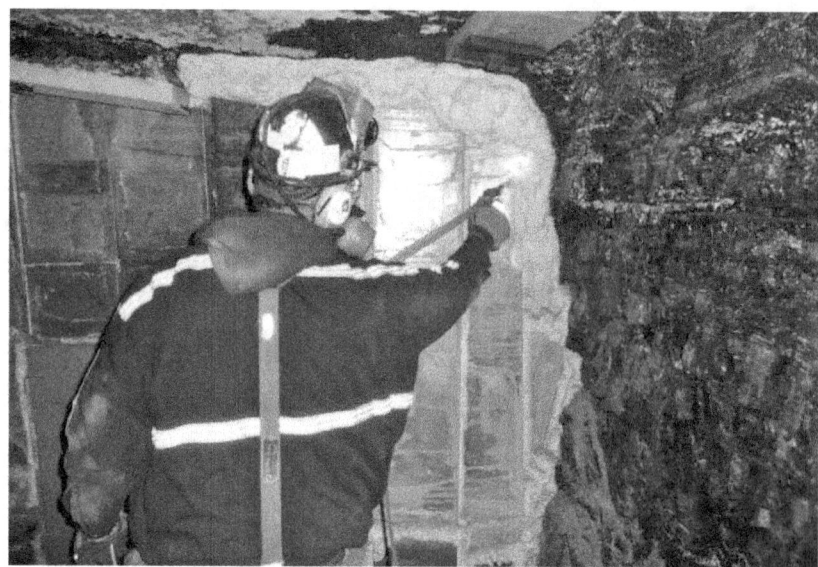

Figure 1. Applying polyurethane foam to a steel ventilation stopping.

Two rock dusters work each shift. One rock duster (called the pod operator) regulates the air pressure at the generator attached to the storage pods while the other (called the hose operator) aims the pressurized hose and applies the rock dust to the mine surfaces. The rock dusters we evaluated traded duties each day. Rock dust, which is primarily calcium carbonate, is applied to the surfaces of the mine to reduce the fraction of combustible material in the mine (Figure 2).

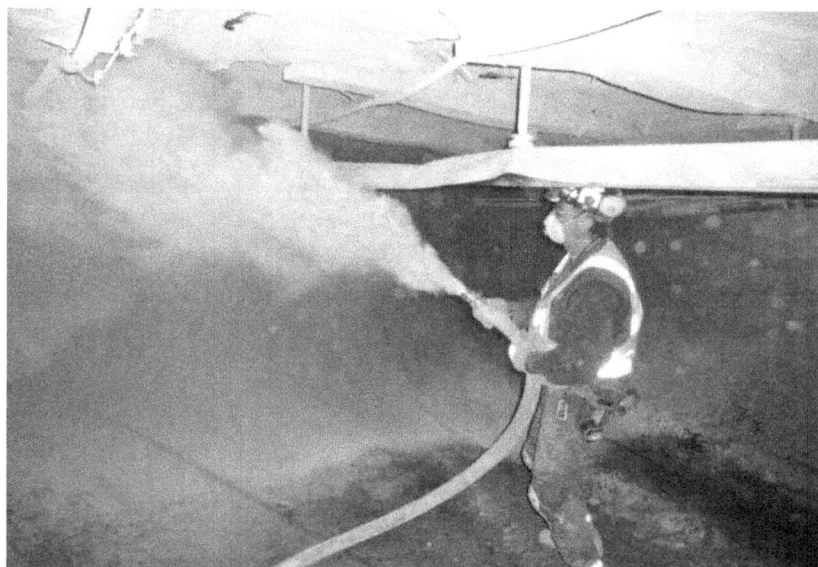

Figure 2. Spraying rock dust onto the surfaces inside the coal mine.

First Evaluation

We did not do air sampling for MDI because aerosols were not generated during the foaming process, and the evaporation of MDI is minimal because of its low vapor pressure (5.4×10^{-6} mmHg at 68°F) [American Plastics Council 1999]. However, we believed that dermal exposure could result from MDI-contaminated equipment or unreacted foam coming into contact with unprotected skin. To evaluate dermal exposure, we sampled the surface of the gun for aromatic isocyanate contamination using Surface Swypes™ (SKC Inc., Eighty Four, Pennsylvania) wipe samples. The foam applicator gun was sprayed with a developer solution and then wiped with a Surface Swype. A second Surface Swype was wiped across the tip of the foam applicator gun where foam material was present (a positive control). A color change to orange or red indicates the presence of aromatic isocyanates.

We collected bulk samples of the rock dust from the storage pods in the mine with a metal spatula and 40-milliliter plastic vials. Two samples each were collected from the storage pods. Half of each sample was analyzed for asbestos using NIOSH Method 9002 [NIOSH 1994]; the other half of each sample was analyzed for silica (specifically quartz) using MSHA Method P-7 [MSHA 1994].

Second Evaluation

Over 3 days, we collected six full-shift PBZ air samples (three from each day-shift rock duster) for respirable dust and silica. Air samples were collected with 37-millimeter sampling cassettes containing preweighed 5-micrometer pore size PVC filters. The filter cassettes were attached to Dorr-Oliver nylon cyclones. AirCheck 2000 pumps (SKC Inc., Eighty Four, Pennsylvania) were used to draw 1.7 liters per minute of air through the sampling media. The Dorr-Oliver nylon cyclones are designed to remove larger particles from the sampled airstream so that the PVC filters collect particles in the size range representative of particles that deposit in the human respiratory tract (i.e., respirable particles). The PVC filters were analyzed for respirable dust using NIOSH Method 0600 [NIOSH 1994] and respirable silica using NIOSH Method 7500 [NIOSH 1994]. In addition, bulk samples from the storage pods were collected daily over the 3-day sampling period and analyzed for silica using NIOSH Method 7500. NIOSH Method 7500 is able to analyze for quartz, crystobalite, and

ASSESSMENT
(CONTINUED)

tridymite. For silica analysis, both the bulk and air samples were pretreated for possible calcite interferences as described in NIOSH Method 7601 [NIOSH 1994].

Appendix A provides information about OELs and potential health effects of the chemicals we evaluated. Table A-1 in the appendix presents the OELs for respirable crystalline silica (quartz).

RESULTS & DICUSSION

MDI Exposures

We found no evidence that bratticemen were exposed to MDI when applying polyurethane foam. The wipe sample taken on the handle of the foam applicator gun was negative, meaning that MDI was ND (< 3 to 5 micrograms/sample). Another wipe sample was collected to determine that the Surface Swypes were capable of detecting MDI. This positive control wipe sample taken across the tip of the foam applicator gun was positive for aromatic isocyanates. Thus, we have confidence that the handle of the gun was not contaminated with MDI.

We reviewed the "Safe Work Instructions" for the Blacksville #2 Mine. According to these instructions, general dilution ventilation, goggles, rubber gloves, and respirators with charcoal filters are required for bratticemen who seal walls with foam. The bratticeman we observed wore light duty (< 0.30 millimeter) nitrile gloves under leather gloves and a North half-mask air purifying respirator (7700-30M) with combination organic vapor cartridges/ P100 particulate filters (75SCP100, North Safety Products, Cranston, Rhode Island). Light duty nitrile gloves have been shown to be effective barriers against polymeric MDI [Society of the Plastics Industry 1994]. Because the handle of the gun was not contaminated with MDI and because the bratticeman wore nitrile gloves when applying foam (including cleaning up and dismantling the foam applicator gun), dermal exposure to MDI appears to be well controlled. Preventing dermal exposure to MDI is important because dermal exposure to isocyanates can lead to skin and respiratory sensitization [Bello et al. 2007].

The combination organic vapor cartridge and P100 filter used with the half-mask air purifying respirator is appropriate for atmospheres containing MDI. These cartridges/filters should be changed out according to a predetermined schedule. The NIOSH and OSHA APF for a half-mask air purifying respirator is 10 [29 CFR 1910.134], which means that inhalable concentrations are expected to be one tenth the ambient concentrations, provided the respirator is worn, maintained, and fitted according to OSHA regulations [29 CFR 1910.134]. Because MDI has a low vapor pressure (5.4 x 10^{-6} mmHg at 68°F) and the foam is injected and not sprayed (which could generate MDI aerosols), we expect that PBZ concentrations of MDI during foam application should be below the NIOSH REL (50 $\mu g/m^3$) or ceiling limit (200 $\mu g/m^3$) [NIOSH 2005]. Therefore, we did not do air sampling.

Asbestos, Respirable Silica, and Respirable Dust Exposures

The rock dust used in the Blacksville #2 Mine is supplied by the Greer Lime Company (Riverton, West Virginia) and according to the January 2008 quality control report, is composed primarily of calcium carbonate (98%), but does contain other compounds including silica (0.75%). The bulk samples we collected did not contain asbestos but did contain crystalline silica (quartz) at levels ranging from ND (< 0.5%) to 0.98% (Table 1). For the bulk samples analyzed by NIOSH Method 7500, only quartz was found; crystobalite and tridymite were not detected.

Table 1. Percent by mass of crystalline silica (quartz) in the bulk samples of rock dust

Sample date	No. of samples	% crystalline silica	Comments
3/31/2009	4	0.4	The bulk samples were collected on the same day and analyzed for quartz using MSHA Method P-7 [MSHA 1994].
9/14/2009 to 9/17/2009	3	ND (< 0.5%) to 0.94	Each bulk sample was collected on a different day and analyzed for quartz, crystobalite, and tridymite using NIOSH Method 7500 [NIOSH 1994]. Crystobalite and tridymite were not detected.

Table 2 provides the air sampling results for respirable dust and crystalline silica. The reported concentrations were time weighted averaged over 8 hours. The respirable dust concentrations were below the OELs for calcium carbonate. Because crystalline silica is more hazardous than calcium carbonate, the crystalline silica sampling results were used to determine safe levels of exposure.

RESULTS AND DISCUSSION
(CONTINUED)

Only quartz, a form of crystalline silica, was found in the air samples; cristobalite and tridymite (other forms of crystalline silica) were not detected. Respirable crystalline silica was present at PBZ concentrations above the MDC of 6 µg/m³ but below the MQC of 25 µg/m³. Because the MQC is equal to the ACGIH TLV, any PBZ concentrations of respirable crystalline silica above the ACGIH TLV would have been quantifiable. Concentrations between the MDC and MQC are listed in Table 2 but are contained within parentheses to point out that there is more uncertainty associated with these values than with concentrations above the MQC.

Table 2. Personal breathing zone air concentrations of respirable dust and crystalline silica for rock dusters measured on the second evaluation

Sample day	Job duty	Respirable dust* (µg/m³)	Respirable silica[†] (µg/m³)
1	Pod operator	250	ND[§]
	Hose operator[‡]	370	(20)
2	Pod operator	430	ND[§]
	Hose operator	1300	(13)
3	Pod operator	360	(12)
	Hose operator	1500	(12)

*Respirable dust concentrations may be compared to OSHA PEL and NIOSH REL for calcium carbonate (5000 µg/m³) [NIOSH 2005].

[†]Respirable silica concentrations may be compared directly to the NIOSH REL of 50 µg/m³ [NIOSH 2005] and ACGIH TLV of 25 µg/m³ [ACGIH 2009]. Values in parentheses represent trace concentrations of respirable silica above the MDC of 6 µg/m³ but below the MQC of 25 µg/m³.

[‡]The hose operator on sample day 1 was exposed to the highest percentage of silica in the respirable dust (5.4%). At this percentage of silica, the OSHA PEL for respirable dust is 1350 µg/m³ [NIOSH 2005], and the MSHA PEL is 1850 µg/m³ [30 CFR 71.1010].

[§]ND = nondetectable (less than the MDC of 6 µg/m³)

The sampling pump worn by the rock duster who operated the hose on the third sample day stopped working for 30 minutes. This happened during a period of time when we perceived the airborne dust to be at higher levels. Consequently, the reported PBZ concentrations of respirable dust and crystalline silica on that day may underestimate the actual concentrations. Furthermore, although the PBZ concentrations of respirable crystalline silica (quartz) were below applicable OELs during this evaluation (see Table A-1 in the appendix), we cannot be certain that rock dusters would not be overexposed at other times. The six air samples we collected may not be representative of the true exposure distribution (e.g., exposures over an entire year) and may not be sufficient to identify an overexposure.

To address the uncertainty of whether an overexposure to crystalline silica may exist, we statistically analyzed the data we collected using IHDataAnalyst V1.01 (Exposure Assessment Solutions Inc.) to approximate the exposure distribution and determine the probability of overexposure. For this analysis, employees were considered overexposed if the 95th percentile of their true exposure distribution was greater than the ACGIH TLV of 25 µg/m³. Hence, exceeding the ACGIH TLV more than 5% of the time (i.e., 5 out of 100 workdays) constitutes an overexposure. Maximum likelihood estimation was used for assigning values to the ND concentrations. According to this analysis, there is a 73% probability that rock dusters are overexposed to respirable crystalline silica. Probability calculations are influenced by sample size and variability within the sample. A larger sample size with less variability leads to tighter confidence intervals and hence smaller probabilities of overexposure. However, collecting more air samples does not always result in less variability.

We used the ACGIH TLV in our statistical analysis because the ACGIH TLV is more protective than the other OELs (see Table 1 in the appendix), and according to a NIOSH health hazard review of occupational exposure to respirable crystalline silica [NIOSH 2002], several epidemiologic studies have found significant risks of silicosis over working lifetimes at concentrations below the current NIOSH REL, OSHA PEL, and MSHA PEL. The ACGIH TLV is intended to prevent pulmonary fibrosis, which may be a risk factor for lung cancer [ACGIH 2006].

According to the Blacksville #2 Mine "Safe Work Instructions," rock dusters are to "apply rock dust in a manner that carries dust away from [them] and wear a respirator." The rock dusters we observed wore half-mask N95 filtering facepiece respirators (2300N95, Moldex®, Culver City, California) during spraying. The NIOSH and OSHA APF for this type of respirator is 10 [29 CFR 1910.134], which means that the inhalable concentrations are expected to be one tenth the ambient concentrations, provided the respirator is worn, maintained, and fitted according to OSHA regulations [29 CFR 1910.134]. Taking into account the protection afforded by this respirator, the probability of exceeding the ACGIH TLV 5% of the time becomes 0.1%. Thus, half-mask N95 filtering facepiece respirators should provide adequate protection from respirable silica exposures. On one occasion when the airflow was stagnant, the rock duster operating the hose wore a PAPR equipped with a helmet (Airstream AS-600-LBC, 3M, St. Paul, Minnesota) and high efficiency particulate filter (3M, AS-140-25). The airborne rock dust concentration appeared higher during this time. This type of respirator has a NIOSH and OSHA APF of 25 [29 CFR 1910.134], and thus provides greater protection than a half-mask respirator.

Although respirators are used at the Blacksville #2 Mine and required for certain operations including foam application and rock dusting, the Blacksville #2 Mine has no comprehensive written respiratory protection program. At the time of this evaluation, employees wearing respirators were not medically evaluated and approved to wear respirators nor were they fit-tested.

CONCLUSIONS

The bratticemen applying polyurethane foam are protected from dermal exposures to MDI because they wear nitrile gloves and because the foam applicator gun was not contaminated with MDI. Inhalation exposures to MDI are unlikely because MDI does not readily evaporate at ambient temperatures in the mine, and the foam is not aerosolized. Asbestos was not found in bulk samples of the rock dust, but crystalline silica (quartz) was found. Although the rock dusters' PBZ concentrations of respirable crystalline silica were below applicable OELs, according to a statistical analysis, there is a 73% probability that their PBZ concentrations may exceed the ACGIH TLV (25 μg/m^3) 5% of the time.

RECOMMENDATIONS

Based on our findings, we recommend the actions listed below to create a more healthful workplace. We encourage the Consolidation Coal Company to use a labor-management health and safety committee or working group to discuss the recommendations in this report and develop an action plan. Those involved in the work can best set priorities and assess the feasibility of our recommendations. Our recommendations are based on the hierarchy of controls approach discussed in the appendix. This approach groups actions by their likely effectiveness in reducing or removing hazards. In most cases, the preferred approach is to eliminate hazardous materials or processes and install engineering controls to reduce exposure or shield employees. Until such controls are in place, or if they are not effective or feasible, administrative measures and/or personal protective equipment may be needed.

Elimination and Substitution

Elimination or substitution of a toxic/hazardous process material is a highly effective means for reducing hazards. Incorporating this strategy into the design or development phase of a project, commonly referred to as "prevention through design," is most effective because it reduces the need for additional controls in the future. Because silica is a naturally occurring mineral, its elimination from rock dust may not be feasible. Similarly, isocyanates are always used in polyurethane foams, and we are not aware of other types of foams that do not contain isocyanates (e.g., latex foams) being used in underground coal mines.

Engineering Controls

Engineering controls reduce exposures to employees by removing the hazard from the process or placing a barrier between the hazard and the employee. Engineering controls are very effective at protecting employees without placing primary responsibility of implementation on the employee.

1. Ensure that airflow is directed to carry rock dust particles away from the rock dusters.

Administrative Controls

Administrative controls are management-dictated work practices and policies to reduce or prevent exposures to workplace hazards. The effectiveness of administrative changes in work practices for controlling workplace hazards depends on management commitment and employee acceptance. Regular monitoring and reinforcement is necessary to ensure that control policies and procedures are not circumvented in the name of convenience or production.

1. Conduct periodic air monitoring to ensure that the respirators employees are using are sufficiently protective or can be eliminated once other controls are in place that reduce PBZ concentrations of silica to acceptable levels.

Personal Protective Equipment

PPE is the least effective means for controlling employee exposures. Proper use of PPE requires a comprehensive program, and calls for a high level of employee involvement and commitment to be effective. The use of PPE requires the choice of the appropriate equipment to reduce the hazard and the development of supporting programs such as training, change-out schedules, and medical assessment if needed. PPE should not be relied upon as the sole method for limiting employee exposures. Rather, PPE should be used until engineering and administrative controls can be demonstrated to be effective in limiting exposures to acceptable levels.

1. Continue to require that bratticemen wear nitrile gloves when applying polyurethane foam. The nitrile gloves should be discarded after each foam application (which includes cleaning up and dismantling the foam applicator gun) to prevent cross contamination. Metatarsal leather gloves can be worn over the nitrile gloves. However, to prevent cross contamination, the leather gloves should not be worn over bare hands or be used for other work processes. This procedure should be clearly stated in the "Safe Work Instructions." Chapter 9 of the MSHA Coal Mine Health Inspection Procedures Handbook provides more information on protecting employees who apply polyurethane foam [MSHA 2003].

2. Change cartridges and filters used in air purifying respirators according to a predetermined schedule. Refer to the OSHA Respiratory Protection eTool at http://www.osha.gov/SLTC/etools/respiratory/change_schedule.html for more information on respirator change-out schedules.

3. Require the use of respirators that are at least as effective as half-mask N95 filtering facepiece respirators during rock dusting. These respirators, when worn and maintained properly, should adequately protect rock dusters from respirable crystalline silica exposures. Required use of these respirators should be clearly stated in the "Safe Work Instructions."

4. Implement a written respiratory protection program. According to MSHA regulations [30 CFR 56/57.5005], the program must meet the requirements of the American National Standard: Practices for Respiratory Protection ANSI Z88.2-1969 [ANSI 1969], which includes training on the proper wear and maintenance of respirators, medical evaluations to determine that employees are physically able to perform their work while wearing respirators, and respirator fit testing. The NIOSH Guide to Industrial Respiratory Protection at http://www.cdc.gov/niosh/87-116.html and OSHA regulations [29 CFR 1910.134] provide additional guidance on implementing a comprehensive written respiratory protection program.

REFERENCES

ACGIH [2006]. Silica, crystalline: α-quartz and crystobalite. In: Documentation of the threshold limit values and biological exposure indices. Cincinnati, OH: American Conference of Governmental Industrial Hygienists.

ACGIH [2009]. Threshold limit values for chemical substances and physical agents and biological exposure indices. Cincinnati, OH: American Conference of Governmental Industrial Hygienists.

American Plastics Council [1999]. MDI/polymeric MDI emissions reporting guidelines for the polyurethane industry. Arlington, VA: Alliance for the Polyurethanes Industry, American Plastics Council [http://www.americanchemistry.com/s_acc/bin.asp?SID=1&DID=5941&CID=1556&VID=]. Date accessed: January 2010.

ANSI [1969]. American national standard: practices for respiratory protection. New York: American National Standards Institute, Inc. ANSI Z88.2-1969.

Bello D, Herrick CA, Smith TJ, Woskie SR, Streicher RP, Cullen MR, Liu Y, Redlich CA [2007]. Skin exposure to isocyanates: reasons for concern. Environ Health Perspect 115(3):328–335.

CFR. Code of Federal Regulations. Washington, DC: U.S. Government Printing Office, Office of the Federal Register.

MSHA [1994]. Quartz analytical method (P-7): infrared dertermination of silica in respirable coal mine dust. Pittsburgh, PA: U.S. Department of Labor, Mine Safety and Health Administration (MSHA).

MSHA [2003]. Coal mine health inspection procedures handbook – chapter 9 – polyurethane foam. In: MSHA handbook series. U.S. Department of Labor, Mine Safety and Health Administration (MSHA) [http://www.msha.gov/readroom/handbook/handbook.html] Date accessed: January 2010.

NIOSH [1994]. NIOSH manual of analytical methods. 4th ed. Schlecht PC, O'Connor PF, eds. Cincinnati, OH: U.S. Department of Health and Human Services, Centers for Disease Control and Prevention, National Institute for Occupational Safety and Health, DHHS (NIOSH) Publication No. 94-113 (August 1994); 1st Supplement Publication 96-135, 2nd Supplement Publication 98-119, 3rd Supplement Publication 2003-154. [http://www.cdc.gov/niosh/nmam].

REFERENCES
(CONTINUED)

NIOSH [2002]. NIOSH hazard review: health effects of occupational exposure to respirable crystalline silica. Cincinnati, OH: U.S. Department of Health and Human Services, Centers for Disease Control and Prevention, National Institute for Occupational Safety and Health (NIOSH) Publication No. 2002-129.

NIOSH [2005]. NIOSH pocket guide to chemical hazards. Barsen ME, ed. Cincinnati, OH: U.S. Department of Health and Human Services, Centers for Disease Control and Prevention, National Institute for Occupational Safety and Health (NIOSH) Publication No. 2005-149.

Society of the Plastics Industry [1994]. Technical bulletin: PMDI user guidelines for chemical protective clothing selection. [http://www.osha.gov/SLTC/autobody/docs/techbjul94.html]. Date accessed: January 2010.

In evaluating the hazards posed by workplace exposures, NIOSH investigators use both mandatory (legally enforceable) and recommended OELs for chemical, physical, and biological agents as a guide for making recommendations. OELs have been developed by Federal agencies and safety and health organizations to prevent the occurrence of adverse health effects from workplace exposures. Generally, OELs suggest levels of exposure that most employees may be exposed up to 10 hours per day, 40 hours per week for a working lifetime without experiencing adverse health effects. However, not all employees will be protected from adverse health effects even if their exposures are maintained below these levels. A small percentage may experience adverse health effects because of individual susceptibility, a preexisting medical condition, and/or a hypersensitivity (allergy). In addition, some hazardous substances may act in combination with other workplace exposures, the general environment, or with medications or personal habits of the employee to produce health effects even if the occupational exposures are controlled at the level set by the exposure limit. Also, some substances can be absorbed by direct contact with the skin and mucous membranes in addition to being inhaled, which contributes to the individual's overall exposure.

Most OELs are expressed as a TWA exposure. A TWA refers to the average exposure during a normal 8- to 10-hour workday. Some chemical substances and physical agents have recommended STEL or ceiling values where health effects are caused by exposures over a short period. Unless otherwise noted, the STEL is a 15-minute TWA exposure that should not be exceeded at any time during a workday, and the ceiling limit is an exposure that should not be exceeded at any time.

In the United States, OELs have been established by Federal agencies, professional organizations, state and local governments, and other entities. Some OELs are legally enforceable limits, while others are recommendations. The U.S. Department of Labor OSHA PELs (29 CFR 1910 [general industry]; 29 CFR 1926 [construction industry]; and 29 CFR 1917 [maritime industry]) are legal limits enforceable in workplaces covered under the Occupational Safety and Health Act. NIOSH RELs are recommendations based on a critical review of the scientific and technical information available on a given hazard and the adequacy of methods to identify and control the hazard. NIOSH RELs can be found in the NIOSH Pocket Guide to Chemical Hazards [NIOSH 2005]. NIOSH also recommends different types of risk management practices (e.g., engineering controls, safe work practices, employee education/training, personal protective equipment, and exposure and medical monitoring) to minimize the risk of exposure and adverse health effects from these hazards. Other OELs that are commonly used and cited in the United States include the TLVs recommended by ACGIH, a professional organization, and the WEELs recommended by the American Industrial Hygiene Association, another professional organization. The TLVs and WEELs are developed by committee members of these associations from a review of the published, peer-reviewed literature. They are not consensus standards. ACGIH TLVs are considered voluntary exposure guidelines for use by industrial hygienists and others trained in this discipline "to assist in the control of health hazards" [ACGIH 2009]. WEELs have been established for some chemicals "when no other legal or authoritative limits exist" [AIHA 2009].

Outside the United States, OELs have been established by various agencies and organizations and include both legal and recommended limits. Since 2006, the Berufsgenossenschaftliches Institut für Arbeitsschutz (German Institute for Occupational Safety and Health) has maintained a database of international

OELs from European Union member states, Canada (Québec), Japan, Switzerland, and the United States available at http://www.dguv.de/bgia/en/gestis/limit_values/index.jsp. The database contains international limits for over 1250 hazardous substances and is updated annually.

Employers should understand that not all hazardous chemicals have specific OSHA PELs, and for some agents the legally enforceable and recommended limits may not reflect current health-based information. However, an employer is still required by OSHA to protect its employees from hazards even in the absence of a specific OSHA PEL. OSHA requires an employer to furnish employees a place of employment free from recognized hazards that cause or are likely to cause death or serious physical harm [Occupational Safety and Health Act of 1970 (Public Law 91–596, sec. 5(a)(1))]. Thus, NIOSH investigators encourage employers to make use of other OELs when making risk assessment and risk management decisions to best protect the health of their employees. NIOSH investigators also encourage the use of the traditional hierarchy of controls approach to eliminate or minimize identified workplace hazards. This includes, in order of preference, the use of: (1) substitution or elimination of the hazardous agent, (2) engineering controls (e.g , local exhaust ventilation, process enclosure, dilution ventilation), (3) administrative controls (e.g., limiting time of exposure, employee training, work practice changes, medical surveillance), and (4) personal protective equipment (e.g., respiratory protection, gloves, eye protection, hearing protection). Control banding, a qualitative risk assessment and risk management tool, is a complementary approach to protecting employee health that focuses resources on exposure controls by describing how a risk needs to be managed. Information on control banding is available at http://www.cdc.gov/niosh/topics/ctrlbanding/. This approach can be applied in situations where OELs have not been established or can be used to supplement the OELs, when available.

Undergound Coal Mines

MSHA has regulatory authority in underground coal mines. Thus, exposures must be maintained below MSHA PELs if they exist for the compounds of interest. Some OELs are more protective or based on more recent scientific information than other OELs. Below we discuss all OELs pertinent to this evaluation, as well as the potential health effects from exposure to the chemicals we evaluated.

Isocyanates

Respiratory sensitization and occupational asthma are the most common adverse health outcomes associated with isocyanate exposure [NIOSH 1978]. Respiratory sensitization can occur at low levels of inhalation exposure [Chan-Yeung 1986]. Hence, the OELs for inhalation exposure to MDI are relatively low (e.g., NIOSH REL is 50 $\mu g/m^3$) [NIOSH 2005]. Evidence suggests that dermal exposure to isocyanates can also lead to skin and respiratory sensitization [Bello et al. 2007]. NIOSH recommends preventing contact of MDI with skin [NIOSH 2005].

Crystalline Silica

Exposure to crystalline silica primarily affects the lungs. Long term exposure can cause pulmonary fibrosis (silicosis) [NIOSH 2005]. According to IARC, inhalation of silica in the form of quartz or cristobalite is considered carcinogenic to humans [IARC 1997], specifically leading to lung cancer. The OELs for respirable crystalline silica (quartz) are provided in Table A-1.

Table A-1. Occupational exposure limits for respirable crystalline silica (quartz)

	OEL (µg/m^3)	Comments
NIOSH REL [NIOSH 2005]	50	For respirable crystalline silica.
OSHA PEL [NIOSH 2005]	10,000 / (% silica + 2)	For respirable dust containing silica. Assuming 100% silica, the OSHA PEL = 98 µg/m^3.
MSHA PEL [30 CFR 71.101]	10,000 / (% silica)	For respirable dust containing silica. Assuming 100% silica, the MSHA PEL = 100 µg/m^3.
ACGIH TLV [ACGIH 2009]	25	For respirable crystalline silica.

Calcium Carbonate

The rock dust is composed primarily of calcium carbonate. No adverse health effects have been found from calcium carbonate exposure [IPCS 1999]. The OSHA PEL and NIOSH REL for calcium carbonate are 5000 µg/m^3 respirable particles [NIOSH 2005]. No specific MSHA PEL or ACGIH TLV exists for calcium carbonate.

References

ACGIH [2009]. Threshold limit values for chemical substances and physical agents and biological exposure indices. Cincinnati, OH: American Conference of Governmental Industrial Hygienists.

AIHA [2009]. AIHA 2009 Emergency response planning guidelines (ERPG) & workplace environmental exposure levels (WEEL) handbook. Fairfax, VA: American Industrial Hygiene Association.

Bello D, Herrick CA, Smith TJ, Woskie SR, Streicher RP, Cullen MR, Liu Y, Redlich CA [2007]. Skin exposure to isocyanates: reasons for concern. Environ Health Perspect 115(3):328–335.

CFR. Code of Federal Regulations. Washington, DC: U.S. Government Printing Office, Office of the Federal Register.

Chan-Yeung M [1986]. Occupational asthma. Clin Rev Allergy 4(3):251–266.

IARC [1997]. Monographs on the evaluation of the carcinogenic risks to humans: silica. Vol. 68. Lyon, France: World Health Organization, International Agency for Research on Cancer [http://monographs.iarc.fr/ENG/Monographs/vol68/volume68.pdf]. Date accessed: January 2010.

IPCS (WHO/International Programme on Chemical Safety) [1999]. International Chemical Safety card: calcium carbonate [http://www.cdc.gov/niosh/ipcsneng/neng1193.html. Date accessed: January 2010.

NIOSH [1978]. NIOSH criteria for a recommended standard: occupational exposure to diisocyanates. Cincinnati, OH: U.S. Department of Health, Education, and Welfare, Health Services and Mental Health Administration, National Institute for Occupational Safety and Health, DHEW (NIOSH).

NIOSH [2005]. NIOSH pocket guide to chemical hazards. Cincinnati, OH: U.S. Department of Health and Human Services, Centers for Disease Control and Prevention, National Institute for Occupational Safety and Health, DHHS (NIOSH) Publication No. 2005-149. [http://www.cdc.gov/niosh/npg/]. Date accessed: January 2010.

This page intentionally left blank.

The Hazard Evaluations and Technical Assistance Branch (HETAB) of the National Institute for Occupational Safety and Health (NIOSH) conducts field investigations of possible health hazards in the workplace. These investigations are conducted under the authority of Section 20(a)(6) of the Occupational Safety and Health Act of 1970, 29 U.S.C. 669(a)(6) which authorizes the Secretary of Health and Human Services, following a written request from any employer or authorized representative of employees, to determine whether any substance normally found in the place of employment has potentially toxic effects in such concentrations as used or found. HETAB also provides, upon request, technical and consultative assistance to federal, state, and local agencies; labor; industry; and other groups or individuals to control occupational health hazards and to prevent related trauma and disease.

The findings and conclusions in this report are those of the authors and do not necessarily represent the views of NIOSH. Mention of any company or product does not constitute endorsement by NIOSH. In addition, citations to websites external to NIOSH do not constitute NIOSH endorsement of the sponsoring organizations or their programs or products. Furthermore, NIOSH is not responsible for the content of these websites. All Web addresses referenced in this document were accessible as of the publication date.

This report was prepared by Kenneth W. Fent and Chad H. Dowell of HETAB, Division of Surveillance, Hazard Evaluations and Field Studies. Health communication assistance was provided by Stefanie Evans. Editorial assistance was provided by Ellen Galloway. Desktop publishing was performed by Robin Smith.

Copies of this report have been sent to employee and management representatives at the Consolidation Coal Company, the Pennsylvania Department of Health, the Occupational Safety and Health Administration Region 3 Office, and the Mine Safety and Health Administration District 2 Office. This report is not copyrighted and may be freely reproduced. The report may be viewed and printed at http://www.cdc.gov/niosh/hhe/. Copies may be purchased from the National Technical Information Service at 5825 Port Royal Road, Springfield, Virginia 22161.

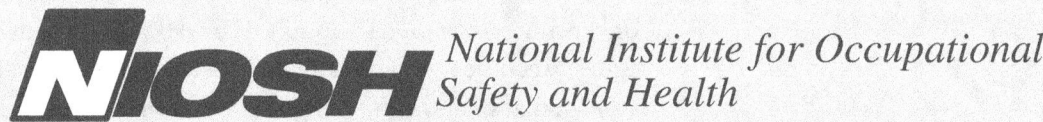

National Institute for Occupational Safety and Health

Delivering on the Nation's promise: Safety and health at work for all people through research and prevention.

www.ingramcontent.com/pod-product-compliance
Lightning Source LLC
Chambersburg PA
CBHW080941290526
45795CB00007BA/2854